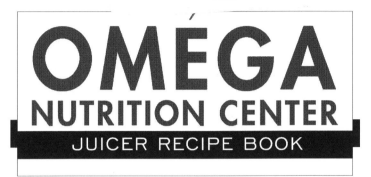

*101 SUPERFOOD JUICE RECIPES FOR ENERGY,
HEALTH AND WEIGHT LOSS!*

BY

SUSAN MICHEL

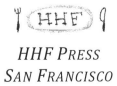

HHF PRESS
SAN FRANCISCO

Legal Notice

The information contained in this book is for entertainment purposes only. The content represents the opinion of the author and is based on the author's personal experience and observations. The author does not assume any liability whatsoever for the use of or inability to use any or all information contained in this book, and accepts no responsibility for any loss or damages of any kind that may be incurred by the reader as a result of actions arising from the use of information in this book. Use this information at your own risk.

The author reserves the right to make any changes he or she deems necessary to future versions of the publication to ensure its accuracy.

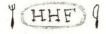

ISBN-13: 978-1539014485
ISBN-10: 1539014487

Published in the United States of America
by Healthy Happy Foodie Press.

www.HHFpress.com

DO YOU LIKE FREE BOOKS?

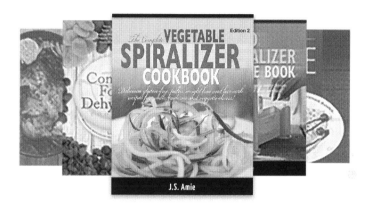

Every month we release a new book, and we offer it to our current readers first...absolutely free! This helps us get early feedback before launching a book, and lets you stock your shelf full of interesting and valuable books for free!

Some recent titles include:

- The Complete Vegetable Spiralizer Cookbook
- My Lodge Cast Iron Skillet Cookbook
- 101 The New Crepes Cookbook

To receive this month's free book, just go to

http://www.healthyhappyfoodie.org/s2-freebooks

Table Of Contents

1

Why You Need This Book!

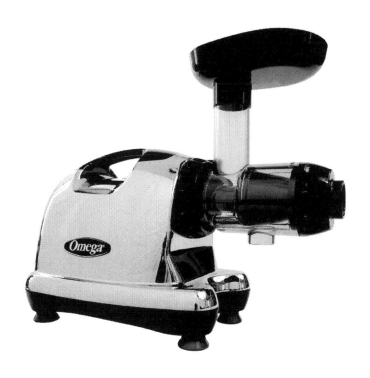

This is The ONLY Juicer Book Written Specifically for Your Omega Juicer

There are many juicing books available today, but this is the only book that will tell you how to make the BEST juice with your superior Omega Juicer. This book explains how to get maximum taste and nutritional benefit from the ingredients you put in your juicer. As you read through this book, you will see why Omega Juicer is not like other juicers. The wide feed chute allows you to juice entire fruits and vegetables, creating nutrition-packed juices. This specially designed chute allows for more variety with easy juicing and clean-up. This book is a must-have and is an important part of owning the Omega Juicer.

Learn How to Combine the Best Ingredients for Flavor and Nutrition

The word "juicing" refers to processing fresh fruit and vegetables with a machine that reduces them to juice and pulp. It is an easy way to consume the foods we need and enjoy their flavor and vitamins. However, did you know that there is a science to combining the right foods, in the right quantities for maximum health benefits?

Learning how to combine these ingredients enables you to create unique flavors, and allows you to mask the flavor of foods that your body needs, but you do not necessarily like. It further allows you to consume superfoods in the proper quantities because you are simply drinking them.

Learn to Make Juice Without the Mess

It has a large capacity pulp container that does not require emptying as often. With less preparation work, there is less to clean-up.

When it is time to clean-up, all parts of Omega Juicer except for the housing are top shelf, dishwasher safe. There is a cleaning brush included to help get particles out of the hard to reach places of the juicing screen or any other parts that may need it.

You Get 101 Great Juice Recipes in One Handy Book

There are enough recipes in this book to last for months. Each and every recipe included has been hand-picked for the Omega Juicer. Some of the characteristics taken into consideration are consistency, nutritional value, and flavor. These recipes have been tested and proven, for the most enjoyable juice. You will find recipes for juices that heal your body. By providing your body with the all-natural vitamins, minerals, and antioxidants it needs; you unleash your body's ability to heal, grow, and regenerate itself.

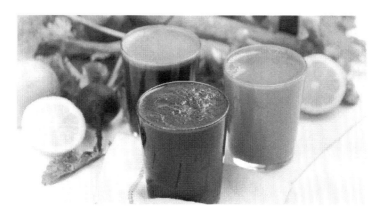

You Get Tips from the Pros

This book provides you with juicing tips from top professionals in the industry. There are tips from medical professionals, chefs, nutritionists, and fitness experts. You will be able to select juices based on flavor and your individual dietary goals.

Whether you are fighting aging, attempting to lose weight or build muscle and enhance energy; the tools you need are as close as your counter top.

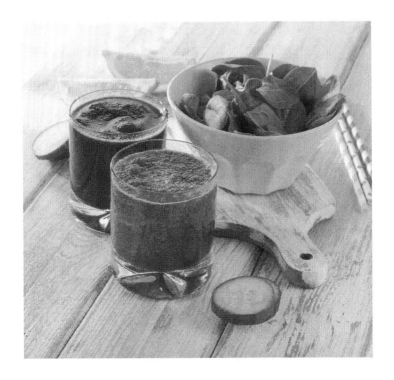

2

Why Choose the Omega Juicer

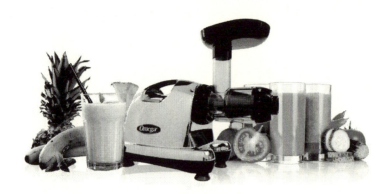

The Omega Juicer is The Absolute Best Way to Make Your Own Juice

The Omega Juicer is a masticating style juicer, which is a type of low-speed juicer. The advantage of this style of juicer is that it protects and maintains many of the nutritious enzymes and prevents oxidation. This will allow you to store your juice for much longer periods of time. The other great aspect of a masticating style juicer is that it more thoroughly extracts the juice from the fruit while allowing much less pulp to find its way into the juice. The result is healthy juice that is free of pulp and seeds.

In addition to the Omega's efficient juice-extracting power, it is also much smaller and lighter than many other commercial-quality juicers. Since fruit and vegetable juice is a great way to get more vital nutrients, having a powerful juicer will ensure that then entire family is getting better nutrition. And since it is so easy to use and clean, you will, no doubt, want to use it every day.

The Omega Juicer Makes More Than Just Juice

If you have purchased an Omega Juicer, you are probably wondering how many different things it can do. The great thing about the Omega Juicer is that it can handle almost any type of fruit or vegetable, and extract the highest amount of juice possible. Part of the secret to making the best possible juice is the addition of the GE Ultem Auger. The auger is the part of the juicer that grinds the produce in order to separate the juice from the solid matter. The Ultem auger is eight times stronger than other plastics and for this reason, it is able to produce a more powerful grind than other juicers. Because of this, you are not limited to simply making juice. The Omega can also make nut butters and pureed fruits and vegetables that can be used as all natural baby foods. You can even use it to make pasta and grind a variety of things like nuts and spices. Once you learn how to take full advantage of your Omega Juicer, the possibilities will be limitless.

The Most Trusted and Durable Juicer on The Market

While it's true that the Omega Juicer is capable of making professional quality juice easily at home, you can also rest assured that you have purchased a juicer that will be durable and dependable in the long term. The Omega juicer is constructed using a high-quality metal housing that can withstand almost anything.

We've already mentioned that the GE Ultem auger is made from the highest quality materials for maximum juice extraction, but much of the reliability of the Omega comes from the low-speed motor that will last for many years and produce the highest quality juice.

The low-speed motor also limits the amount of froth and foam that is often found in homemade juices. This foam is the result of the motor processing the produce too quickly and can produce an unpleasant texture. Because the Omega's motor works at a lower speed, you will always have crisp, clean tasting juice every time.

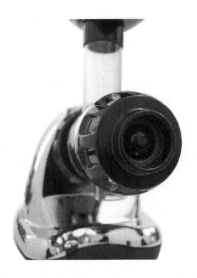

Cleaning The Omega Juicer is Easy and Fast

The Omega Juicer does an amazing job juicing but it's also fast and easy to clean. The components of the juicer come apart easily, and the openings are large enough that cleaning is never challenging. We recommend that you buy a simply bottle brush to clean the inside of the juicer. Since the Omega does an excellent job of containing the leftover produce pulp, you will not need to spend hours trying to get the pulp out of the inside of the juicer. Simply use the brush to clear out any debris that has resulted and rinse with hot water. All of the removable parts of the Omega Juicer are dishwasher safe, but in many cases you will only need to give them a rinse before drying and using again.

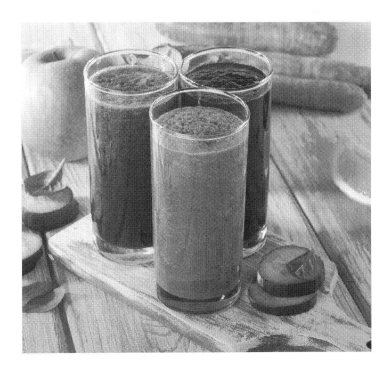

It's The Most Economical Juicer on the Market

Because the Omega uses a two-stage juicing system, you are sure to get the most juice from your produce making the Omega the most efficient and economical juicer on the market. Many juicers use only a single juicing stage where the produce is crushed and juice is collected. If you have ever used a single stage juicer, you have probably noticed that it takes a great deal of produce to make enough juice. The Omega Juicing system, on the other hand, uses two stages to maximize the amount of juice produced.

The Ultem auger is far stronger than many other auger systems, and it allows the Omega to do a much more thorough job of crushing the fruits or vegetables. When the produce is crushed, a certain amount of juice is produced but before the pulp is ejected, the Omega initiates a pressing stage that extracts even more juice from the pulp. It is this second stage that sets the Omega apart from many other comparably priced juicers. You will notice immediately that you are getting more juice every time you use the Omega and that means you are spending less money on your juice. This way, you can afford to use your Omega every day, and enjoy the many health benefits of freshly pressed juice.

3

How to Use Your Omega Juicer

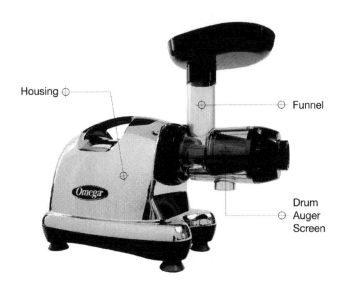

Housing

Funnel

Drum
Auger
Screen

How to Set Up Your Omega Juicer

In order to get the best results from your Omega Juicer, you will want to make sure you have properly set up all of its components. Luckily, this is fast and easy to do regardless of how you are going to use the juicer. The largest part of the Omega juicer is the housing which contains the motor. Place the housing on a level surface and connect the drum to the housing by turning the locking clip clockwise until it is secure. Then place the funnel into the guide at the very top of the drum. After the drum and funnel are in place, insert the auger into the drum. It should fit easily. If you are going to use your Omega to make juice, the next step is to insert the juicing screen into the drum and then secure it in place with the end cap. For non-juicing applications, you will insert the blank attachment into the drum instead of the juicing screen. Finally, place the juice bowl and waste bowl under the drum. These attachments will separately catch the juice and pulp that results from juicing. Once you have completed these steps, simply plug your Omega in and you are ready to juice.

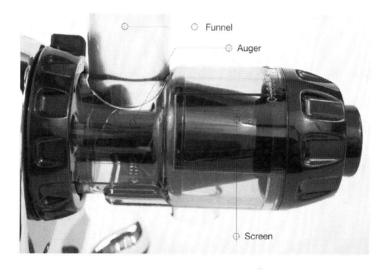

How to Make the Best Fruit and Vegetable Juices

Once you have properly assembled your Omega juicer, you are instantly able to start making the best juice you have ever had, and best of all, it couldn't be easier. Press the ON button and the motor will begin working. Start by placing a few chunks of fruit or vegetables into the funnel and use the plunger to press down gently. Once the fruit reaches the auger inside the housing, you should see juice almost immediately. You can alternate different fruits and vegetables as you juice without changing any attachments or accessories. As you add

21

fruits or vegetables to the juicer, make sure that you allow the juicer to do its job thoroughly. Since the Omega is a low-speed juicer, it is designed to extract the most juice possible from everything you put into it. This means that the Omega employs two separate stages of juicing. The first stage grinds the material which extracts the majority of the juice but the pressing stage ensures that all of the available juice is also extracted from the pulp giving you the best value for your money. Once you have finished juicing, turn off the motor and clean all of the components thoroughly.

How to Use Your Omega to Mince, Chop, and Puree

In addition to juicing and making pasta, your Omega juicer also functions as a powerful food processor. By using the blank attachment and no pasta nozzle you can process a wide variety of foods. You can even grind meat and make healthy, homemade nut butters. To use the Omega to grind, simply assemble it with the blank attachment rather than the juicing screen. Turn on the motor and feed whatever you want to chop into the funnel. The ground material should come out through the spout. If you want a finer grind, you can pass it through the juicer again. To make nut butters you will set up the Omega the same way, but first be sure that the nuts you are using are completely shelled and cleaned. Turn on the motor and feed the nuts into the funnel. When making nut butters you will most likely need to add some canola oil as you add the nuts. This will give the nut butter a smoother texture.

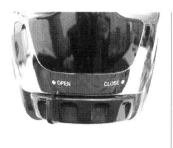 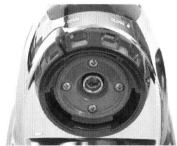

How to Properly Clean and Store Your Omega Juicer

Once you are finished using your Omega juicer, it is important that you properly clean and store it for future use. To clean your Omega, disassemble all of its components and rinse them in warm water. All of the parts except for the housing can be washed in the dishwasher. Before storing your Omega, you will want to make sure that all of the parts are completely dry. Then you can either store it fully assembled or in separate parts.

4

Pro Tips for Juicing

To Remove Toxins, Soak Produce in Water with Vinegar

Your produce can pick up all sorts of harmful microorganisms on its way to your home. The acid in vinegar effectively kill some of those microorganisms. It needs to be in the correct ratio of water to vinegar. You want to use 3 parts water to 1-part vinegar. You can also buy commercial strength vinegar solutions that are more effective. If you're soaking your produce in the sink, make sure to clean your sink thoroughly first.

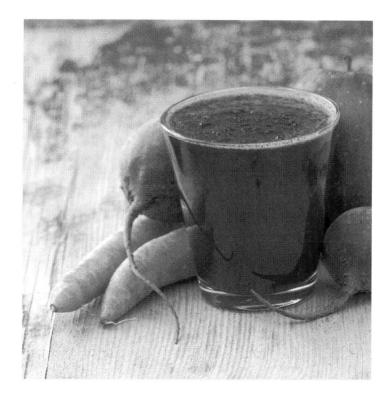

Juice Entire Fruit if Skin is Edible

You may not realize it, but you're losing a lot of nutrients when you peel many of your produce items. Half of the nutrition in an apple is held in its skins. Leaving edible skin will give you a huge amount of nutrients without affecting the flavor.

Remove Large Pits and Seeds Before Juicing

Always remove the hard seeds, stones, and pits from produce like apples, apricots, peaches, etc. They're not easy for the juicer to break down and will cause your juice to breakdown over time. Many of them also contain small amounts of cyanide which can be harmful to your health in large doses.

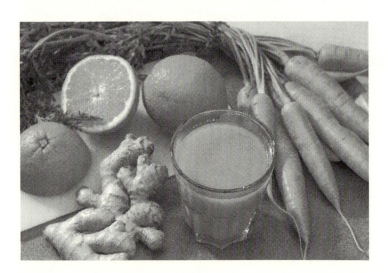

Stringy Vegetables Are Difficult to Juice

For stringy vegetables like spinach, and celery and clog up your juicer. You can help with this problem by alternating your stringy vegetables with a hard vegetable like a carrot. Pre-cutting your stringy vegetables to a quarter inch long also helps.

Always clean your juicer after using it to help keep clogs from forming.

Put in Small Quantities of Greens and Wheatgrass at a Time

Putting in small quantities of these items ensures that the juicer won't get clogged. It will also make it easier to push the items down during the juicing process

Cut Vegetables Up

Cutting vegetables into small pieces ensures that your juicer will run smoothly. Not only will it run smoothly, but you'll ensure that it's able to extract every drop of juice.

5

How to Store Extra (leftover) Juice

Store Leftover Juice in a Glass Container with an Airtight Lid

Glass containers are the best way to store extra juice. You can purchase Mason jars in several sizes which are perfect for various juice needs. Using small (half-jars) are great for taking an extra serving with you in the car. Larger sizes are perfect for juice for the family. The lids are interchangeable.

Fill Containers All the Way to The Top to Keep Air from Reducing Lifespan

You want to avoid allowing air into the jar, so fill the jar to the top and tightly secure the lid. Adding a few drops of lemon juice will keep the juice fresh longer.

Freeze Juice in Freezer Bags or Ice Trays for Easier Access

Again, air is the enemy. Use various sizes of freezer zipper bags to freeze juices. Use a sharpie to label and date the juice.

Freeze in ice trays for fun treats for the children. Adding a popsicle stick makes these juice cubes perfect for a summer treat. Use juice cubes in a different flavor juice for fun and creative flavors.

6

Anti-Aging

Ageless Avocado

Servings: 1 | Prep Time: 1 minute

The only anti-aging super-food, avocado is perfectly balanced and packs a nutritious punch! Combined with the hydrating effects of cucumber, and collagen building lemons, and you have nature's remedy for aging.

Ingredients:

2 cucumbers

1 avocado

1 lemon

Directions:

1.   Peel and pit avocado.

2.   Slice the cucumbers and lemon into small portions.

3.   Using your Omega juicer, place the ingredients into the chute and wait until all is juiced.

4.   Serve with ice and enjoy!

Nutritional Info: Calories: 517 | Sodium: 25 mg | Dietary Fiber: 18.1 g | Total Fat: 40.0 g | Total Carbs: 44.5 g | Protein: 8.4 g.

Beauty with Beets

Servings: 2 | Prep Time: 10 minutes

Beets slow down the age process. They are full of antioxidants and they are a good source of folate, magnesium, iron, potassium, copper as well as vitamin C and B6. Beets help to detoxify the liver and eliminate dead skin cells. The combination of beets with fresh oranges are unexpectedly delicious.

Ingredients:

4 navel oranges

3 red beets

Directions:

1. Peel and seed the navel oranges, dividing into quarters.
2. Scrub and trim the beets.
3. Press the oranges into the food chute with your Omega Juicer followed by the oranges.
4. Stir and pour juice over ice before drinking.

Nutritional Info: Calories: 206 | Sodium: 58 mg | Dietary Fiber: 10.3 g | Total Fat: 0.6 g | Total Carbs: 50.7 g | Protein: 4.7 g.

Beetroot Blush

Servings: 1 | Prep Time: 3 minutes

Turn back the hands of time with this vitamin and mineral packed juice, which is filled with antioxidants. Skin is revived by eliminating dead skin cells. Sagging, dull and splotchy skin is soon repaired leaving a more vibrant and more beautiful complexion.

Ingredients:

1/2 beetroot

1 medium fuji apple

1/2-inch ginger

1 medium lemon

5 leaves lettuce

Directions:

1. Core, deseed, and slice the apple into small chunks.

2. For better juicing, slice all the other ingredients into small portions.

3. Using the pusher, guide the ingredients into the chute of your Omega juicer.

4. Juice the ingredients alternately.

5. Drink and enjoy!

Nutritional Info: Calories: 150 | Sodium: 37 mg | Dietary Fiber: 7.6 g | Total Fat: 0.9 g | Total Carbs: 38.8 g | Protein: 2.4 g.

Kiwi Apple Celery

Servings: 1 | Prep Time: 10 Minutes

Kiwis are a nutritional super fruit. They have 6 times more vitamin C than oranges, and contain phytonutrients that protect DNA from damage. Celery and apples are packed with fiber that moves toxins out of the digestive system.

Ingredients:

1 kiwi

1 apple

1 celery stalk

Directions:

1.	 Peel and slice the kiwi. Cut up the apple and, remove the seeds. Roughly chop the celery stalk.

2.	Using your Omega Juicer, juice the fruits alternately with the celery.

*Nutritional Info: Calories: 144 | Sodium: 18 mg |
Dietary Fiber: 7.0 g | Total Fat: 0.8 g |
Total Carbs: 36.8 g | Protein: 1.5 g.*

Kiwi Grape

Servings: 4 | Prep Time: 12 Minutes

Kiwis have 6 times the vitamin C as oranges. Vitamin C is a powerful antioxidant that will keep many aspects of your body healthy. Grapes contain anti-aging phytonutrients such as resveratrol.

Ingredients:

8 ripe kiwis

2 cups green grapes

2 granny smith apples

1 teaspoon fresh lemon juice

Directions:

1. Peel the kiwis. Slice, core, and remove the seeds from the apples

2. Turn ON your Omega juicer and place the fruits in the chute.

3. Add the lemon juice and serve.

Nutritional Info: Calories: 171 | Sodium: 7 mg |
Dietary Fiber: 7.2 g | Total Fat: 1.1 g |
Total Carbs: 42.8 g | Protein: 2.3 g.

Mango Magic

Servings: 1 | Prep Time: 5 minutes

The magic of mango has been known for centuries for its skin rejuvenating properties. Mango produces collagen and allows natural healing of the skin. Combined with hydrating cucumber, this is a wrinkle fighting formula that leaves your skin with a healthy glow.

Ingredients:

1/2 mango

1 medium cucumber

1/2 lemon

1 cup purslane (or spinach or kale)

Handful cilantro

Directions:

1.   Slice and deseed the mango.

2.   Put all of the ingredients through your Omega Juicer, alternating the harder foods (cucumber, mango, and lemon) with the leafy greens (purslane, cilantro).

Nutritional Info: Calories: 139 | Sodium: 51 mg |
Dietary Fiber: 5.8 g | Total Fat: 1.0 g |
Total Carbs: 32.8 g | Protein: 4.5 g.

Pomegranate Apple

Servings: 2-3 | Prep Time: 15 Minutes

Pomegranates contain a huge amount of antioxidant that fight free radicals that cause aging. Pectin in the apples helps remove toxins from the digestive tract.

Ingredients:

2 medium to large apples

2 medium to large pomegranates

Directions:

3. Core and deseed apples then, slice the apples into small portions. Cut up the pomegranate and remove the seeds.

4. Place the fruits one by one in the chute. Use the pusher when needed.

Nutritional Info: Calories: 195 | Sodium: 2 mg | Dietary Fiber: 5.4 g | Total Fat: 0.3 g | Total Carbs: 51.1 g | Protein: 1.5 g.

Purple Rain

Servings: 1 | Prep Time: 2 minutes

This purple juice hydrates your skin with cucumber, while fighting wrinkles with the power of blackberries this juice is rich in antioxidants that keep the skin looking healthy and young. Blackberries carry anthocyanins that stimulate the body's production of collagen and elastin.

Ingredients:

2 cups of blackberries

1 cucumber

1 stalk of celery

1 green apple

Directions:

1. Trim the white ends of the celery. Slice the cucumber; core and deseed apples.

2. Place the ingredients in the chute of your Omega juicer. Juice the hard fruits alternately with the softer ones.

3. This is a juice that can be served over ice and garnished with lemon if you choose.

Nutritional Info: Calories: 266 | Sodium: 24 mg | Dietary Fiber: 21.4 g | Total Fat: 2.1 g | Total Carbs: 64.2 g | Protein: 6.6 g.

Radiant Raspberry-Avocado

Servings: 2 | Prep Time: 6 minutes

Raspberries rejuvenate the skin and reverse skin cell damage. Add them to the anti-aging super-food, avocado and oranges (for collagen production) and ageing has met its match.

Ingredients:

1 avocado

1 large (or 2 medium) oranges

1 1/2 cups raspberries

Directions:

1. Peel and pit the avocado. Peel the oranges and remove the seeds. Place the fruit into the chute of the Omega juicer.

2. Using the food pusher, push the fruit into the juicer.

*Nutritional Info: Calories: 296 | Sodium: 7 mg |
Dietary Fiber: 14.9 g | Total Fat: 20.3 g |
Total Carbs: 30.5 g | Protein: 3.9 g.*

Raspberry Orange Banana

Servings: 1 | Prep Time: 10 Minutes

Raspberries contain lots of compounds that fight aging such as quercetin, gallic acid, and ellagic acid. The oranges are high in Vitamin C which helps with collagen production.

Ingredients:

2 oranges, peeled and segmented

60g fresh raspberries

1 medium banana, peeled

3 fresh mint leaves

Directions:

1.   Peel the banana. Peel and rip the oranges into segments.
2.   Juice all ingredients with the mint leaves.

Nutritional Info: Calories: 311 | Sodium: 3 mg | Dietary Fiber: 16.0 g | Total Fat: 1.2 g | Total Carbs: 77.6 g | Protein: 5.6 g.

Scarlett Sunset Glow

Servings: 4 | Prep Time: 8 minutes

When we nourish our bodies on the inside; it shows on the outside. This mineral and vitamin packed juice slows aging and gives your skin a youthful and radiant glow. The cucumber hydrates the cells, while the oranges aid in restoring collagen and elasticity to the skin. The addition of beetroot is essential to restore the structure of skin cells.

Ingredients:

1 beetroot

1 stick of celery

2 medium red apples

2 carrots

1 cucumber

2 oranges

Directions:

1. Peel and quarter the oranges. If you do not like an earthy taste, you may remove the celeriac from the beet root.

2. If you have an aversion to beetroot, you may substitute any dark berry of your choice; beginning with one cup and adding more to taste.

3. Slice, core, and deseed the other ingredients into small portions.

4. Juice the ingredients, using Omega juice, in order listed.

5.   Use the pulp for your soup or just add them in your compost.

*Nutritional Info: Calories: 122 | Sodium: 46 mg |
Dietary Fiber: 6.0 g | Total Fat: 0.4 g |
Total Carbs: 30.8 g | Protein: 2.2 g.*

Very Berry Juice

Servings: 1 | Prep Time: 5 Minutes

The berries in the juice have lots of antioxidants and anti-inflammatory compounds that will help keep your body young. The Pectin in apples helps with both digestive, and heart health.

Ingredients:

2 apples

1 cucumber

1 handful of blueberries

1 handful of strawberries

1 handful of raspberries

1 handful of blackberries

Directions:

1. Slice the apples and cucumber into small portions.

2. Slowly place the fruits in your Omega juicer. Do not overfill the chute.

3. Juice by batches or alternately.

Nutritional Info: Calories: 362 | Sodium: 12 mg | Dietary Fiber: 21.3 g | Total Fat: 2.2 g | Total Carbs: 91.5 g | Protein: 5.7 g.

7

Heart

Antiox-Orange

Servings: 2 | Prep Time: 10 Minutes

The produce in the juice are high in various antioxidants that help the heart. It also helps to improve eye health with its high content of carotenoids.

Ingredients:

4 small oranges

6 carrots

3 cucumbers

2 yellow bell peppers (capsicum)

2-inch piece of ginger

Directions:

1. Peel and slice the ingredients into small portions.

2. Alternately juice the ingredients using your Omega juicer.

Nutritional Info: Calories: 322 | Sodium: 145 mg | Dietary Fiber: 15.8g | Total Fat: 2.0 g | Total Carbs: 74.8 g | Protein: 8.8 g.

Crazy Cranberry

Servings: 1 | Prep Time: 5 Minutes

Cranberries improve vascular function, and blood pressure. It also helps to lower bad cholesterol.

Ingredients:

1 cup (230 g) fresh cranberries

1 – 2 large oranges

5 carrots

Directions:

1. Peel the oranges.
2. Juice the carrots alternately with the oranges and cranberries.

Nutritional Info: Calories: 423 | Sodium: 210 mg | Dietary Fiber: 24.7 g | Total Fat: 0.4 g | Total Carbs: 94.2 g | Protein: 6.0 g.

8

Liver

Kidney Health

Servings: 2 | Prep Time: 7 Minutes

Parsley and cucumbers have been shown to help and even prevent kidney stones. Carotenoids in carrots are great for detox.

Ingredients:

1 large cucumber

3 stalks of celery

1 ounce of parsley

3 medium to large carrots

Directions:

1. Prepare ingredients: Peel and slice carrots and cucumber, wash and cut parsley into small portions.

2. Juice the ingredients in order listed or alternately (hard fruits and greens).

Nutritional Info: Calories: 69 | Sodium: 94 mg | Dietary Fiber: 3.9 g | Total Fat: 0.3 g | Total Carbs: 16.1 g | Protein: 2.3 g.

Liver Tonic

Servings: 1 | Prep Time: 7 Minutes

The carrots are alkalizing which will help get rid of toxins from the liver. They're also packed with liver healthy vitamin A. Beets contain betaine which aids in digestion, and helps to detox and health the liver. Apples contain pectin which binds to toxins before they get to your liver.

Ingredients:

1 large apple

4 carrots

1 beet

Directions:

1. Slice, core and remove the seeds from the apple.
2. Slice the carrots and beet into small portions.
3. Juice all ingredients on your Omega Juicer.

Nutritional Info: Calories: 260 | Sodium: 247 mg | Dietary Fiber: 13.4 g | Total Fat: 0.6 g | Total Carbs: 64.8 g | Protein: 4.3 g.

9

Bones and Joints

Joint Juice

Servings: 3 | Prep Time: 8 minutes

Sore and painful joints are soothed almost instantly with this powerful drink. Loaded with vitamins and minerals as well as potent anti-inflammatory properties, this juice relieves painful joints even for people with conditions such as arthritis.

Ingredients:

1 apple

3 carrots, large

4 asparagus spears

1 broccoli stalk

3/4 cups parsley

1 tablespoon extra-virgin olive oil

Directions:

1. Pour the tablespoon of Olive Oil directly into the juicer jug. Do NOT put Olive Oil through the Omega Juicer. Use Extra Virgin Olive Oil and do not substitute other oils.

2. Peel and slice carrots; wash and cut the greens into small portions.

3. Feed the fruits and vegetables through the Omega juicer.

Nutritional Info: Calories: 129 | Sodium: 72 mg |
Dietary Fiber: 5.7 g | Total Fat: 5.1 g |
Total Carbs: 20.6 g | Protein: 3.5 g.

Popeye Juice

Servings: 2 | Prep Time: 10 Minutes

Spinach and apples are both high in bone building calcium. Grapefruit has been shown to slow down bone loss.

Ingredients:

1 1/2 cups spinach

1/2 grapefruit, peeled, white pit removed

2 green apples, cut into eighths

1 (1-inch) piece fresh ginger, peeled

2 large stalks celery

Directions:

1. Peel the grapefruit. Slice the apples, core them, and remove the seeds. Peel the ginger.

2. Turn ON your Omega juicer and place the ingredients one by one. Juice the ingredients, serve, and enjoy!

Nutritional Info: Calories: 124 | Sodium: 71 mg | Dietary Fiber: 6.4 g | Total Fat: 0.6 g | Total Carbs: 31.2 g | Protein: 1.9 g.

Terrific Turmeric

Servings: 1 | Prep Time: 5 minutes

This is your "go to" recipe for painful joints and inflammation. Every ingredient in this juice packs a pain killing and inflammation reducing PUNCH! The crowning glory in this cocktail is turmeric. Turmeric is super-powerful and it contains more anti-inflammatory properties than perhaps any other food.

Ingredients:

1 cucumber

3 carrots

1 bunch of celery

1 1/2 inches of turmeric root

1-inch ginger root

2 cups pineapple

Directions:

1. Peel and slice the ingredients.

2. Place the fruits in the chute of your Omega juicer. Juice them by batches or by not overfilling the chute.

3. Drink immediately. Any leftover juice should be stored in an airtight container, in the refrigerator and consumed within 48 hours.

Nutritional Info: Calories: 324 | Sodium: 179 mg | Dietary Fiber: 13.1 g | Total Fat: 1.6 g | Total Carbs: 79.7 g | Protein: 6.3 g.

The Green Team

Servings: 1 | Prep Time: 2 minutes

When it comes to healthy bones, watercress is an excellent food choice. Watercress provides a massive amount of calcium and vitamin K which is great for the bones as well as the clotting factors of the blood. This juice has a zesty and tangy flavor.

Ingredients:

3 ounces (1 bunch) watercress

1 lime

2 celery stalks

2 green apples

Directions:

1. Peel, core, and deseed apples. Slice apples and lime into small portions.

2. Feed the ingredients into the chute of the Omega Juicer. Start juicing with apples, watercress, celery, and then lime.

Nutritional Info: Calories: 232 | Sodium: 84 mg | Dietary Fiber: 12.3 g | Total Fat: 1.3 g | Total Carbs: 58.6 g | Protein: 4.2 g.

10

Constipation

Berry Dandelion Spice

Servings: 1 | Prep Time: 3 minutes

This spicy and zesty drink is great for fighting constipation. This fiber rich drink carries is super-charged with antioxidants and Vitamin C. It will relieve your bloating discomfort while boosting your immune system and heart health.

Ingredients:

1 cup dandelion leaves

1 small chili

1 cup raspberries

1 cup strawberries

1/2 teaspoon alcohol-free stevia

Directions:

1. Remove the placental skin and seed of the chili. Process all foods through the Omega chute. Juice the greens in between the berries.

2. Stir and serve.

3. Note, if your berries are sweet, you may omit the stevia. Use more or less chili according to taste. This drink may be served over ice.

Nutritional Info: Calories: 141 | Sodium: 71 mg |
Dietary Fiber: 28.3 g | Total Fat: 1.9 g |
Total Carbs: 31.5 g | Protein: 4.2 g.

11

Detox

Apple Cinnamon

Servings: 1 | Prep Time: 7 Minutes

Apples help to flush out both the liver and the kidneys. Cinnamon has anti-inflammatory compounds.

Ingredients:

3 apples, cored and cut into large pieces – small enough to fit into the juicer

1/2 teaspoon ground cinnamon

Directions:

1. Run the apples into the Omega Juicer chute.
2. Mix in the cinnamon.

Nutritional Info: Calories: 287 | Sodium: 5 mg | Dietary Fiber: 13.8 g | Total Fat: 1.0 g | Total Carbs: 76.3 g | Protein: 1.5 g.

Beet Carrot Apple Dandelion Green

Servings: 1 | Prep Time: 10 Minutes

The dandelion greens are great for liver health. The beet aid with cleansing the blood, and is packed with vitamins and minerals. The carrots and apples contain lots of antioxidants

Ingredients:

1 cup dandelion greens

1 small beet

3 carrots

1 apple

Directions:

1. Slice up the apples and remove the seeds. Peel and quarter the beet. Slice the carrots and de-stem the dandelion.

2. Run the dandelion greens in between apple, carrots, and beet.

Nutritional Info: Calories: 216 | Sodium: 208 mg | Dietary Fiber: 11.8 g | Total Fat: 0.8 g | Total Carbs: 53.2 g | Protein: 4.3 g.

Beetroot Pomegranate

Servings: 1 | Prep Time: 10 Minutes

Pomegranates are super foods high in antioxidants. They also have antiviral properties, and can help lower blood pressure. Beetroot is high in vitamins B and C, and helps to detox the liver and blood.

Ingredients:

3 normal sized beetroots

5-6 blood oranges

2 red apples

1 large pomegranate

Directions:

1. Peel the beetroots, and the oranges. Slice the apples and remove the seeds. Cut up the pomegranate and remove the seeds and juice. Discard the peel and white membrane.

2. Alternate running the soft and hard produce through your Omega juicer.

Nutritional Info: Calories: 766 | Sodium: 80 mg | Dietary Fiber: 33.9 g | Total Fat: 1.9 g | Total Carbs: 194.3 g | Protein: 12.3 g.

Calming Citrus Cleanse

Servings: 1 | Prep Time: 10 minutes

Pineapples contain bromelain which aids in digestion. Oranges are high in vitamin C and antioxidants. Ginger has great anti-inflammatory properties.

Ingredients

1/4 pineapple

2 oranges

1/2 lime

1 knob of ginger

Directions:

1. Peel the oranges, and pineapple. Slice the pineapple and lime.
2. Wash the ginger thoroughly.
3. Juice the ingredients on your Omega juicer.

Nutritional Info: Calories: 376 | Sodium: 16 mg | Dietary Fiber: 16.4 g | Total Fat: 3.3 g | Total Carbs: 88.4 g | Protein: 8.2 g.

Carrot Apple Juice

Servings: 10 ounces | Prep Time: 5 Minutes

Carrots are packed with vitamins and minerals especially vitamin A. Vitamin A helps your liver flush out toxins. Apples have a huge amount of antioxidants and can even help reduce your risk of cancer.

Ingredients:

3 or 4 carrots

1 granny smith apple

Directions:

1. Cut the apple into pieces and remove the seeds.

2. Place all ingredients in your Omega juicer alternating between pieces of apple and carrots.

Nutritional Info: Calories: 97 | Sodium: 85 mg | Dietary Fiber: 5.2 g | Total Fat: 0.2 g | Total Carbs: 24.6 g | Protein: 1.2 g.

Clean Green Juice

Servings: 1 | Prep Time: 2 minutes

Detox your body with "Clean Green Juice". This cocktail is a natural diuretic promoting kidney health. Loaded with vitamins, this juice is great for the skin. You will look and feel amazing. You will reboot your system with massive supplies of vitamins, minerals and nutrients, including magnesium, folate, iron, copper and potassium.

Ingredients:

1/2 cucumber

1 stalk celery

10 leaves spinach

1/2 cup parsley

Directions:

1. Wash and slice cucumber and celery. De-stem spinach and parsley.

2. Using your Omega juicer, run the greens in between cucumber and celery.

3. You may garnish this with a slice of lemon (optional). Drink and enjoy!

Nutritional Info: Calories: 19 | Sodium: 19 mg |
Dietary Fiber: 1.1 g | Total Fat: 0.2 |
Total Carbs: 4.0 g | Protein: 1.1 g.

Dandy Dandelion Detox

Servings: 1 | Prep Time: 8 minutes

This dandelion-kale juice is loaded with nutrient rich vitamins and minerals such as iron, copper, magnesium. This will allow you to reach your goal of eating enough vegetables while assisting your body to naturally detox. Drink this juice first thing in the morning, before eating. The dandelion is a natural diuretic which will restore your body's water balance. This works well with the hydrating properties of cucumber. The added nutritional value of kale and spinach will all your maximum nutritional benefits while detoxing. You will heal your body from the inside out with the benefits of cucumber, celery and lemon.

Ingredients:

3 handfuls of spinach

1/2 bunch of dandelion greens

1/2 bunch kale

1/2 cucumber

4 carrots

4 stalks of celery

1 lemon

1-inch piece of ginger

Directions:

1. Wash thoroughly and slice ingredients from cucumber down to ginger. De-stem greens.
2. Juice the greens in between hard ingredients.

3.   You may add a pinch of cayenne pepper for garnish or a pinch of sea salt to spice up the flavor.

Nutritional Info: Calories: 346 | Sodium: 630 mg |
Dietary Fiber: 22.1 g | Total Fat: 2.5 g |
Total Carbs: 73.2 g | Protein: 21.2 g.

Detox Boost

Servings: 1 | Prep Time: 10 Minutes

Spicy lemongrass helps to remove built up toxins and aids in digestion. Lime helps increase alkalinity, and move along the detox process. Watermelon is hydrating which will help clear toxins from the system.

Ingredients:

3 cups watermelon

1/2 stalk lemongrass

1 lime

1-inch piece of ginger

Directions:

1.   Wash, and slice ginger and lime, about half an inch. Cut watermelon into cubes.

2.   Juice the ingredients using your Omega juicer. Juice lemongrass in between other ingredients.

Nutritional Info: Calories: 208 | Sodium: 11 mg |
Dietary Fiber: 4.3 g | Total Fat: 1.2 g |
Total Carbs: 53.3 g | Protein: 4.2 g.

Dynamic Duo

Servings: 1 | Prep Time: 1 minute

This simple juice combo carries some serious power. These two ingredients can help lower cholesterol and blood pressure, while providing the body with minerals and fiber.

Ingredients:

3 carrots

1 granny smith apple

Directions:

1.   Core and deseed apple. Slice carrots into small portions.

2.   Feed the chute of your Omega juicer slowly until all ingredients are juiced.

3.   Enjoy this juice in seconds!

Nutritional Info: Calories: 170 | Sodium: 128 mg | Dietary Fiber: 8.9 g | Total Fat: 0.3 g | Total Carbs: 43.1 g | Protein: 2.0 g.

Florida Detox Juice

Servings: 1 | Prep Time: 5 minutes

If you are looking for a sunny, citrus juice that will allow you to detox in the most flavorful way, this is the juice for you. Get the detoxing effect of grapefruit, oranges and lemons with the skin rejuvenating properties of collagen-building vitamin C. This juice can be used as a daily cleanse to remove unwanted toxins from your body. This juice leaves taste buds tingling with sour lemon, tart grapefruit and sweet oranges.

Ingredients:

1 lemon

1 grapefruit

2 oranges

Directions:

1. Peel grapefruit and oranges. The peel can be removed from the lemon or left on for additional nutritional benefits or removed.

2. If peel is intact on lemon, use the food pusher to move it down the chute of your Omega Juicer.

3. Then, juice grapefruit and oranges. It could not be easier. You are ready to enjoy your delicious juice.

Nutritional Info: Calories: 228 | Sodium: 1 mg | Dietary Fiber: 11.6 g | Total Fat: 0.7 g | Total Carbs: 58.2 g | Protein: 4.8 g.

Glorious Green Juice

Servings: 1 | Prep Time: 5 minutes

This glorious green juice provides tons of nutrients that promote the body's natural detoxification process. Nutritionists agree that getting huge amounts of phytonutrients is the best way to reboot the system. This juice optimizes nutritional benefits during detox.

Ingredients:

2 green apples

1 cucumber

4 kale leaves

1 cup parsley

1 head of broccoli

1-inch of ginger

1-inch piece of jalapeno pepper

Directions:

1. Slice the fruits into small portions, about half an inch.
2. Run all the greens in between the fruits.
3. Turmeric is a good garnish for this juice.

Nutritional Info: Calories: 311 | Sodium: 79 mg | Dietary Fiber: 15.6 g | Total Fat: 2.1 g | Total Carbs: 75.9 g | Protein: 8.1 g.

Granny's Groovy Green Juice

Servings: 1 | Prep Time: 6 minutes

This sweet little recipe is extra flavorful, due to the delicious Granny Smith apples. Combined with the super-food, kale and some zesty lemon this is one of the most flavorful way to detox. This is a power packed juice that will leave you refreshed and energized.

Ingredients:

4 granny smith apples

3 stalks celery

2 leaves kale

4 cups spinach

1 lemon

Directions:

1. Slice the fruits and de-stem the greens.

2. Process kale, spinach, and lemon through your Omega Juicer, in between celery and apples.

Nutritional Info: Calories: 433 | Sodium: 145 mg | Dietary Fiber: 22.8 g | Total Fat: 2.0 g | Total Carbs: 112.1 g | Protein: 6.5 g.

Green Apple Zest

Servings: 1 | Prep Time: 3 minutes

This juice is light and refreshing. The crisp apple and tangy lemon juice is recommended for detoxification, but could become a summertime, family favorite. This easy to drink juice has fiber-rich apples and hydrating cucumber. The citric acid found in lemon, aides in digestion.

Ingredients:

1 lemon

2 green apples

1 cucumber

1/2 cup of cold water

Directions

1. Add 1/2 cup cold water to the juice jug.
2. Peel, Core and deseed apples. Slice cucumber and lemon.
3. Run the lemon through the food chute with the Omega Juicer.
4. Press the green apples and cucumber down the chute.
5. Stir vigorously and drink.

Nutritional Info: Calories: 252 | Sodium: 14 mg | Dietary Fiber: 12.0 g | Total Fat: 1.2 g | Total Carbs: 66.8 g | Protein: 3.6 g.

Inner Glow

Servings: 1 | Prep Time: 5 Minutes

The cucumbers are high in minerals and hydrating. The added hydration will help you expel toxins. The basil is antimicrobial, antifungal, anti-inflammatory, and antiviral. Lime is alkalizing and will balance out your pH.

Ingredients:

1 cucumber

1 apple

1/2 lime

1 small handful basil

Ingredients:

1. Cut up the apple and remove the seeds. Peel the lime.
2. Juice the lime, and basil alternately with the cucumber and apple.

Nutritional Info: Calories: 152 | Sodium: 9 mg | Dietary Fiber: 7.0 g | Total Fat: 0.8 g | Total Carbs: 39.8 g | Protein: 3.0 g.

Kiwi Orange Juice

Servings: 1 | Prep Time: 5 Minutes

This juice has a ton of vitamin C from both fruits. Oranges contain a lot of antioxidants. This juice also increases iron absorption.

Ingredients:

3 kiwis

2 oranges

Directions:

1. Wash the kiwis well, and cut away the peel of the oranges doing your best to keep the white pith. The pith contains many antioxidants.

2. Juice the ingredients on your Omega juicer.

Nutritional Info: Calories: 312 | Sodium: 7 mg | Dietary Fiber: 15.7 g | Total Fat: 1.6 g | Total Carbs: 76.7 g | Protein: 6.1 g.

Strawberry-Carrot Apple Juice

Servings: 2 | Prep Time: 5 minutes

This juice is made with strawberries, carrots, apples and cucumber. This is like visiting a farmer's market. Packed with flavor and fiber and loaded with nutrients, it is the perfect detox juice. This juice removes toxins and leaves you feeling fantastic. This juice is also popular with children.

Ingredients:

1 large cucumber

1 large red apple

2 medium carrots

6 large strawberries

Directions:

1. Prepare ingredients by slicing into small portions. Core and deseed apple.
2. Turn "ON" your Omega juicer and start to run the ingredients into the chute.

Nutritional Info: Calories: 106 | Sodium: 46 mg | Dietary Fiber: 5.2 g | Total Fat: 0.4 g | Total Carbs: 26.8 g | Protein: 2.0 g.

The Toxin Killer

Servings: 2 | Prep Time: 7 Minutes

The ingredients in this juice are packed with antioxidant. It's great daily juice to keep your body free of toxins.

Ingredients:

3 apples

1 stick of celery

Half a cucumber

1 handful spinach

1 handful lettuce

Directions:

1.   Cut up the apple and remove the seeds. Slice the celery and cucumber. Wash and peel off the leaves of greens.

2.   Juice the spinach and lettuce in between cucumber, celery, and apples.

Nutritional Info: Calories: 182 | Sodium: 74 mg |
Dietary Fiber: 9.3 g | Total Fat: 1.0 g |
Total Carbs: 45.7 g | Protein: 3.8 g.

Watermelon Cucumber juice

Servings: 4 | Prep Time: 10 Minutes

Watermelon and cucumber are both hydrating, and help the body get rid of toxins. Limes help to alkalize the body and regulate pH.

Ingredients:

1/2 (4 pound) watermelon

4 cucumbers

2 limes

Directions:

1. Cut the watermelon into cubes, and remove the seed. Peel the limes. Slice the cucumbers.

2. Juice the ingredients using your Omega juicer by placing them one by one in the chute.

Nutritional Info: Calories: 123 | Sodium: 10 mg | Dietary Fiber: 3.3 g | Total Fat: 0.7 g | Total Carbs: 31.5 g | Protein: 3.5 g.

12

Immune System

Apple Beet

Servings: 4 | Prep Time: 15 Minutes

The vitamin C, iron, folate, phytochemicals, and manganese in beets all help to boost the immune system. Apples (red) contain quercetin which helps to fortify and boost the immune system.

Ingredients:

3 medium beets

10 – 15 apples

Directions:

1. Cut up the beets. Slice the apples and remove the seeds.
2. Juice the beets, and apples on your Omega juicer.

Nutritional Info: Calories: 383, Sodium: 54 mg, Dietary Fiber: 17.8 g, Total Fat: 1.3 g, Total Carbs: 100.5 g, Protein: 2.9 g.

Cantaloupe Orange

Servings: 1 | Prep Time: 10 Minutes

Cantaloupe and oranges are both high in immune boosting vitamin C. Cantaloupe is also high in carotenoids which stop free radicals from harming your body.

Ingredients:

1/4 Cantaloupe

1 Orange

Dash of cinnamon

Directions:

1. Peel the orange. Slice up the cantaloupe, making sure to keep the rind on.

2. Feed the cantaloupe and orange into Omega juicer chute. Use the food pusher to press on the fruits.

3. Mix in the cinnamon.

Nutritional Info: Calories: 99 | Sodium: 6 mg | Dietary Fiber: 4.9 g | Total Fat: 0.3 g | Total Carbs: 24.7 g | Protein: 2.0 g.

Ginger Turmeric Shots

Servings: 7 | Prep Time: 10 minutes

These small shots pack a cold fighting punch. Ginger, and turmeric have strong antibacterial, and antimicrobial compounds that will help fight off colds and flus. Lemons contain immune boosting vitamin C.

Ingredients:

1 apple

2 lemons

2-inch piece of ginger root

2-inch piece of turmeric root

Directions:

1. Slice the apple, core it, and remove the seeds. Peel the turmeric, and lemons; slice them.

2. Feed the Omega chute with the ingredients and enjoy it in seconds!

Nutritional Info: Calories: 31 | Sodium: 2 mg | Dietary Fiber: 1.7 g | Total Fat: 0.4 g | Total Carbs: 7.5 g | Protein: 0.5 g.

Immune Enhancer

Servings: 2 | Prep Time: 10 Minutes

This juice contains more than 100% of your daily dose of immune boosting vitamins A & C. Vitamin C helps to boost the immune system by killing free radicals. Vitamin A is an anti-infective, which means it fights invading organisms and infections.

Ingredients:

1 lemon

2 cm slice of ginger

3 medium carrots

4 stalks of celery

4 kiwi fruit

A handful of parsley

Directions:

1. Slice the ingredients to fit the Omega chute.

2. Juice the ingredients. Run the parsley in between the hard ingredients.

Nutritional Info: Calories: 186 | Sodium: 139 mg |
Dietary Fiber: 11.0 g | Total Fat: 1.8 g |
Total Carbs: 42.4 g | Protein: 5.6 g.

Orange Aloe Vera

Servings: 1 | Prep Time: 12 Minutes

Oranges are packed with Vitamin C which boosts the immune system and can help your body fight off a cold. Aloe vera contain bradykinase which stimulate the immune system, and fights infection.

Ingredients:

3 organic oranges

2 fresh aloe vera branches

Directions:

1. Peel the oranges. Slice the top skin off the aloe vera and then the sides. The gel will be at the bottom. Remove it and discard the rest of the aloe vera.

2. Juice the oranges on your Omega juicer.

3. Place the aloe and juice in a blender and blend on low speed until combined.

Nutritional Info: Calories: 261 | Sodium: 9 mg | Dietary Fiber: 13.2 g | Total Fat: 0.7 g | Total Carbs: 65.4 g | Protein: 5.2 g.

Peach Medley

Servings: 4 | Prep Time: 12 Minutes

Peaches have a large amount of ascorbic acid, and zinc. Both help to boost and support the immune system. Zinc also improves wound healing.

Ingredients:

2 large apples

10 medium carrots

1/2 lemon

1 large orange

2 large peaches

Directions:

1. Cut up the apples and remove the seeds. Cut up the peaches and remove the pit. Peel the lemon and orange.

2. Juice the ingredients in your Omega juicer.

Nutritional Info: Calories: 175 | Sodium: 106 mg | Dietary Fiber: 8.9 g | Total Fat: 0.5 g | Total Carbs: 43.9 g | Protein: 2.8 g.

The Immune Shot

Servings: 1 | Prep Time: 10 Minutes

This juice is packed with the typical immune supporting vitamin A & C. It's also high in vitamin B6 which help the body produce anti-bodies. The spinach is high in iron which play a vital role in immune health. Ginger helps fight infections.

Ingredients:

1 medium bunch of celery (or one package of celery hearts)

1 fuji apple (or other bold, sweet and crispy apple of choice)

1/2 of a lime

1 cup spinach

1 cup kale

1 piece of fresh ginger (about the size of a gum ball)

Directions:

1. Peel the lime and slice, about half an inch. Slice, core, and remove the seeds from the apple.

2. Juice the ingredients using your Omega juicer. Juice the greens in between other ingredients.

Nutritional Info: Calories: 161 | Sodium: 88 mg | Dietary Fiber: 8.0 g | Total Fat: 0.8 g | Total Carbs: 40.0 g | Protein: 4.1 g.

Turbo Express

Servings: 1 | Prep Time: 10 Minutes

Spinach is high in iron which helps boost the immune system. Pineapple is high in Vitamin C which helps boost the immune system, and helps fight off colds.

Ingredients:

2 apples

A handful of spinach leaves

1 slice of cucumber

1 slice of lime

Half a celery stick

1/4 pineapple

1/4 avocado

Direction:

1. Slice the apples, core them, and remove the seeds. Slice cucumber, lime, and celery. Cube the pineapple.

2. Juice the ingredients by running the spinach in between other produce.

3. Place the juice in a blender with the avocado until well mixed.

Nutritional Info: Calories: 399 | Sodium: 178 mg | Dietary Fiber: 18.8 g | Total Fat: 11.6 g | Total Carbs: 77.0 g | Protein: 9.9 g.

13

Eyes

Cantaloupe Carrot

Servings: 1 | Prep Time: 10 Minutes

Cantaloupe and carrots are both rich in carotenoids. Carotenoids help prevent macular degeneration, and cataracts.

Ingredients:

1/4 cantaloupe

2 large carrots

Directions:

1. Slice up the cantaloupe, keeping the rind on.
2. Juice both the cantaloupe and carrots on your Omega juicer.

Nutritional Info: Calories: 71 | Sodium: 105 mg | Dietary Fiber: 3.9 g | Total Fat: 0.1 g | Total Carbs: 17.0 g | Protein: 1.5 g.

Carrot Celery Bell Pepper

Servings: 1 | Prep Time: 7 Minutes

The carrots and bell peppers are both high in carotenoids that keep eyes healthy. Carrots also contain vitamin A which helps protect the surface of the eye. Bell peppers contain lutein which helps prevent cataracts and macular degeneration.

Ingredients:

4 carrots

2 celery stalks

1/2 a red bell pepper

Directions:

1.   Cut up the bell pepper.

2.   Juice all ingredients on your Omega juicer.

Nutritional Info: Calories: 124 | Sodium: 198 mg | Dietary Fiber: 7.8 g | Total Fat: 0.2 g | Total Carbs: 28.6 g | Protein: 2.8 g.

14

Beauty

Carrot Apple Mint

Servings: 1 | Prep Time: 10 Minutes

Carrots are high in both vitamins A&C which helps with boost collagen, normalize skin function, and fight acne. The complex vitamin profile found in all 3 ingredients will also give you energy, and boost your metabolism.

Ingredients:

5 carrots

1 apple (red delicious ideally)

1 cup mint loosely packed

Directions:

1. Cut up the apples and remove the seeds. De-stem mints.

2. Alternately juice apple and mints using your Omega jucier.

Nutritional Info: Calories: 260 | Sodium: 239 mg |
Dietary Fiber: 18.1 g | Total Fat: 1.0 g |
Total Carbs: 62.8 g | Protein: 6.0 g.

Cucumber Lemon Avocado

Servings: 2 | Prep Time 10 Minutes

The fatty acids in avocado will help your skin looks its best. Cucumbers are very hydrating and will do the same for you skin, giving it a nice glow.

Ingredients:

2 cucumbers (peeled)

1 lemon (peeled)

1 avocado (peeled and seeded)

Directions:

1. Peel the lemon. Slice cucumber, and peel and seed the avocado.

2. In your Omega juicer, juice and cucumbers.

3. Place the juice and avocado in a blender and blend on high until liquid. The avocado will not juice well in a juicer.

*Nutritional Info: Calories: 259 | Sodium: 13 mg |
Dietary Fiber: 9.1 g | Total Fat: 20.0 g |
Total Carbs: 22.3 g | Protein: 4.2 g.*

Glowing Skin

Servings: 4 | Prep Time: 7 Minutes

Beetroot helps heal and prevent acne. Carrots are high in vitamin A which helps to normalize skin. Oranges are high in vitamin C which aids in collagen productions, reduce scarring, and helps give skin a natural glow. Cucumbers are hydrating which will help flush the skin of toxins.

Ingredients:

1 beetroot

2 oranges

2 carrots

2 red apples

1 cucumber

1 stick of celery

Directions:

1. Slice the apples and remove the seeds. Cut up the beetroot. Peel the oranges.

2. Feed the ingredients one by one in the chute. Enjoy your healthy juice in seconds!

Nutritional Info: Calories: 121 | Sodium: 36 mg | Dietary Fiber: 5.9 g | Total Fat: 0.4 g | Total Carbs: 30.5 g | Protein: 2.1 g.

Passionate Pink Juice

Servings: 1 | Prep Time: 5 minutes

Every ingredient in this juice is flavorful, packed with minerals, and vitamins and hand chosen to make you beautiful. The minerals and folate in beets are consumed worldwide for their anti-aging properties. They are essential for beautiful skin, hair and to slow the effects of aging. The bioactive compounds in ginger assists in having a sharp mind and an efficient body. It is known for its anti-nausea benefits but ginger is also a great food for skin tone and reducing the appearance of scars. Pear and pineapple are both fruits that will give you a glowing complexion.

Ingredients:

1 beet

1 cup pineapple

1-inch ginger

1 pear

Directions:

1. Slice/Cut the ingredients in to small chunks. Deseed pear.

2. Place ingredients into the chute of your Omega Juicer and press through with the food pusher. This pretty pink juice can be served over ice if you choose.

Nutritional Info: Calories: 224 | Sodium: 82 mg |
Dietary Fiber: 9.2 g | Total Fat: 0.9 g |
Total Carbs: 56.3 g | Protein: 3.5 g.

Pineapple- Spinach Juice

Servings: 1 | Prep Time: 5 Minutes

This refreshing juice will help keep your skin glowing. Pineapple contains vitamin C which aids in collagen formation and may help reverse dark spots. Romaine has a ton of vitamin A which helps aid in normalizing skin function. No matter what problems you have with your skin this juice can help.

Ingredients:

1 cup baby spinach

5 cups chopped romaine

3 cups chopped pineapple

Directions:

1. Slice the pineapple and greens, about half an inch.
2. Juice the greens in between the sliced pineapples.

Nutritional Info: Calories: 258 | Sodium: 32 mg | Dietary Fiber: 7.6 g | Total Fat: 0.8 g | Total Carbs: 67.0 g | Protein: 3.9 g.

Tomato Vegetable

Servings: 1 | Prep Time: 10 Minutes

Parsley helps balance sebum production and works to detox the liver. Tomatoes are high in vitamin C which helps with dark spots, scarring and collagen production.

Ingredients:

2 large tomatoes

1 stalk celery

1 cucumber

1 handful of fresh parsley

1/2 teaspoon pink Himalayan sea salt

Pinch of cayenne pepper

Handful of ice

Directions:

1. Cut up the tomatoes and slice the celery.
2. Juice in your Omega the tomatoes, celery, parsley, and cucumber alternately.
3. Place the juice in a shaker cup with the cayenne, salt, and ice.
4. Shake until all ingredients are well mixed.

Nutritional Info: Calories: 168 | Sodium: 121 mg | Dietary Fiber: 11.2 g | Total Fat: 2.3 g | Total Carbs: 35.2 g | Protein: 9.8 g.

Watermelon Guava

Servings: 3 | Prep Time: 10 Minutes

Watermelon and guava are both high in vitamins A&C, as well as the antioxidant lycopene. These nutrients are skin vitamins. Vitamin A works to normalize skin, and reduce pore size, while lycopene gets rid of free radicals that can cause wrinkles.

Ingredients:

2 cups chilled watermelon

1 cup chilled guava juice

2 teaspoons lemon juice

1/2 teaspoon salt

Directions:

1. Cut the watermelon into cubes.

2. Using Omega juicer, juice the watermelon.

3. Combine all the ingredients in a pitcher, and stir until well mixed.

4. Garnish with watermelon balls if desired.

Nutritional Info: Calories: 69 | Sodium: 39 mg | Dietary Fiber: 3.4 g | Total Fat: 0.7 g | Total Carbs: 15.6 g | Protein: 2.0 g.

15

Fiber Rich

Blackberry Kiwi

Servings: 1 | Prep Time: 15 Minutes

Blackberries, kiwi, and pineapple are all high in fiber. Fiber helps remove toxins from your digestive track. Kiwi also protects DNA from being damaged.

Ingredients:

1/4 large pineapple, peeled, cored and cut into cubes

1 cup blackberries

1 kiwifruit, peeled

1 pear

30 fresh mint leaves

Directions

1. Prepare the ingredients—Peel and core pineapple, wash blackberries, peeled and slice kiwifruit, core and deseed pear, and de-stem mint

2. Little by little, feed the chute with the ingredients. Juice the mint in between fruits.

Nutritional Info: Calories: 208 | Sodium: 9 mg | Dietary Fiber: 15.3 g | Total Fat: 1.4 g | Total Carbs: 50.9 g | Protein: 3.9 g.

Heart Beet

Servings: 4 | Prep Time: 5 Minutes

Lemons, apples, and beets all help relieve constipation. Additionally, beets help to detox liver, and both lemons and oranges help the body to become more alkaline.

Ingredients:

1 apple

1 beet

12 carrots

1/2 lemon

2 oranges

Directions:

1. Peel the oranges. Cut the apple into slices and take out the seeds. Slice the carrots and lemon.

2. Juice the ingredients in your Omega juicer.

Nutritional Info: Calories: 155 | Sodium: 146 mg |
Dietary Fiber: 8.5 g | Total Fat: 0.3 g |
Total Carbs: 38.3 g | Protein: 3.0 g.

Pear Celery Lemonade

Servings: 1 | Prep Time: 10 Minutes

Celery and pears are packed with digestive healthy fiber. The lemons and pears also contain a lot of antioxidant rich vitamin C. Add in the optional chia seeds if you're looking for even more fiber.

Ingredients:

2 pears, peeled and cored

2 to 3 large juicy lemons, peel and pith removed

3 stalks celery

1 tablespoon chia seeds (optional)

Directions:

1. Peel and core the pears. Remove the peel and pith from the lemons. Slice the celery.

2. Gradually fill the chute and use the pusher to juice.

3. Add in the chia seeds if using, and stir. Allow the juice to rest in the refrigerator for 10-15 until the chia seeds have plumped up.

Nutritional Info: Calories: 284 | Sodium: 48 mg |
Dietary Fiber: 17.0 g | Total Fat: 1.0 g |
Total Carbs: 76.0 g | Protein: 3.1 g.

Pineapple Cucumber Refresher

Servings: 2 | Prep Time: 5 Minutes

This juice has a sweet flavor from the pineapple, and is quite refreshing because of the cucumber. Cucumbers are very hydrating thanks to their high water content.

Ingredients:

2 large slices of pineapple

1 1/2 large red apple

1/2 cucumber

1/2 lemon

Directions:

1. Slice the pineapple, and quarter and seed the apples.

2. Juice all produce in your Omega juicer.

Nutritional Info: Calories: 105 | Sodium: 3 mg |
Dietary Fiber: 4.9 g | Total Fat: 0.4 g |
Total Carbs: 27.8 g | Protein: 1.1 g.

The Digestive Helper

Servings: 1 | Prep Time: 5 Minutes

Grapefruits are great for both blood pressure, and heart health. Bromelain in pineapple aids in digestion. Lemons help with digestion as well, and can kick start your metabolism especially in the morning.

Ingredients:

1/4 pineapple

1 yellow grapefruit

1 ruby grapefruit

1 lemon

1 carrot

Directions:

1. Cut up and peal the pineapple
2. In your Omega juicer, run all the ingredients alternately. Serve and enjoy!

Nutritional Info: Calories: 146 | Sodium: 44 mg |
Dietary Fiber: 6.6 g | Total Fat: 0.5 g |
Total Carbs: 38.0 g | Protein: 3.0 g.

The Eye Opener

Servings: 3.5 | Prep Time: 5 Minutes

Apples contain a natural laxative that's helped by the addition of the carrots. The vitamin A & C in the apples, and antioxidants improve skin health.

Ingredients:

2 oranges

2 apples

14 carrots

Directions:

1. Peel the oranges, cut the apple into slices and discard the seeds.

2. Enjoy juicing with your Omega juicer by feeding the chute with your ingredients.

Nutritional Info: Calories: 204 | Sodium: 169 mg | Dietary Fiber: 11.0 g | Total Fat: 0.3 g | Total Carbs: 50.7 g | Protein: 3.3 g.

Watermelon Chia Juice

Servings: 2 | Prep Time: 5 Minutes

The chia seeds are packed with fiber, omega 3's, and energy boosting nutrients. The watermelon is hydrating. The lime is rich in vitamin C, and the mint gives it a nice flavor.

Ingredients:

6 cups watermelon

1 sprig of mint leaves

1/2 lime

1 heaping tablespoon of chia seeds

Directions:

1. Cube the watermelon, and remove the skin from the lime.

2. Juice the mint in between watermelon and lime.

3. Place the juice on a pitcher with the chia seeds and stir. Let the juice rest in the refrigerator for 10-15, until the chia seeds plump up.

Nutritional Info: Calories: 172 | Sodium: 11 mg | Dietary Fiber: 5.1 g | Total Fat: 4.0 g | Total Carbs: 41.6 g | Protein: 4.8 g.

16

Digestion

Digest Ease Juice

Servings: 1 | Prep Time: 10 Minutes

The fennel helps the body to get rid of excess fluids and stops excess gas from building up. Apples contain pectin which helps keep food moving. Ginger helps with gas, and can sooth an upset stomach.

Ingredients:

1/2 to 1-inch piece of ginger

1/4 to 1/2 of a large fennel bulb (about 4 ounces)

3 carrots

1 apple

2 celery stalks with leaves

Directions:

1. Cut up the fennel bulb. Chop the apples, and remove the seeds. Slice the celery and ginger.

2. Use your favorite Omega juicer. Remember to juice the hard and soft ingredients alternately.

Nutritional Info: Calories: 228 | Sodium: 215 mg | Dietary Fiber: 13.6 g | Total Fat: 0.9 g | Total Carbs: 56.0 g | Protein: 4.1 g.

Digest Zest Juice

Servings: 1 | Prep Time: 10 Minutes

Ginger helps relax booth the small and large intestine. It also helps to get rid of excess gas. Pineapple contains bromelain which helps to break down food.

Ingredients:

2 cups of chopped pineapple, include the cores

1/2 lime or lemon, peeled

2 apples, peeled if not organic

1/2-inch ginger root

1 tablespoon apple cider vinegar (optional)

Direction:

1. Chop up the pineapple. Chop the apples and remove the seeds. Peel the lemon or lime.

2. Juice the sliced ingredients in your Omega juicer.

3. Add in the apple cider vinegar if using, and stir.

Nutritional Info: Calories: 374 | Sodium: 9 mg | Dietary Fiber: 14.7 g | Total Fat: 1.3 g | Total Carbs: 99.2 g | Protein: 3.3 g.

17

Anti-Inflammatory

Mango Pear Spinach

Servings: 1 | Prep Time: 10 Minutes

Mangos contain proteolytic enzymes that fight inflammation. Spinach has phytonutrients that have anti-inflammatory affects as well.

Ingredients:

2 pears

1 mango

1 cup spinach

Directions:

1. Cut up and core the pear. Slice the mango and spinach, about 1/2-inch.

2. Altogether, juice the ingredients in your Omega juicer.

Nutritional Info: Calories: 394 | Sodium: 33 mg | Dietary Fiber: 17.4 g | Total Fat: 1.3 g | Total Carbs: 99.9 g | Protein: 3.4 g.

Orange Turmeric

Servings: 2 | Prep Time: 10 Minutes

Turmeric is one of the most powerful natural anti-inflammatory foods. Oranges contain compounds that decreases the development of inflammatory joint conditions.

Ingredients:

4 oranges peeled

4 large carrots

2-inch piece of turmeric skin removed

Directions:

1. Peel the oranges, and the turmeric.
2. Juice the oranges in order listed using your Omega juicer.

Nutritional Info: Calories: 250 | Sodium: 101 mg | Dietary Fiber: 13.4 g | Total Fat: 0.9 g | Total Carbs: 60.7 g | Protein: 5.0 g.

Strawberry Pear Coconut Water

Servings: 1 | Prep Time: 10 Minutes

This juice has a triple threat of anti-inflammatory produce. Pears have anti-inflammatory phytonutrients, ginger contains anti-inflammatory compounds, and helps digestion, and strawberries lowers C-reactive protein which is a marker of inflammation.

Ingredients:

3 cups fresh organic strawberries, stems removed

1 organic pear, cored and seeded

1/4 fresh lime

Small piece of ginger

1/2 cup coconut water

Directions:

1.   Remove the stems from the strawberries. Slice the pear, core and deseed it. Peel and slice the lime and ginger.
2.   Feed all ingredients in your Omega juicer.
3.   Mix the juice with coconut water.

Nutritional Info: Calories: 382 | Sodium: 16 mg |
Dietary Fiber: 17.6 g | Total Fat: 15.2 g |
Total Carbs: 65.5 g | Protein: 5.3 g.

The Ranch Mocktail

Servings: 4 | Prep Time: 7 Minutes

Cantaloupe and ginger are both chalked full of anti-inflammatory compounds. Cantaloupe also has a wide spectrum of antioxidants, and ginger aids in digestion. Try this drink as a healthy alternative to a cocktail.

Ingredients:

1 whole cantaloupe

2 celery stalks

1 apple

1/4-inch piece of ginger

1 (750ml) bottle of sparkling water

Salt to taste

Directions:

1. Cut up the cantaloupe. Slice the apple and remove the seeds.
2. Juice all the produce on your Omega juicer.
3. In a pitcher mix the sparkling water and juice. Salt to taste.
4. Serve immediately.

Nutritional Info: Calories: 39 | Sodium: 15 mg | Dietary Fiber: 1.6 g | Total Fat: 0.2 g | Total Carbs: 9.7 g | Protein: 0.5 g.

18

General Health Support

Beet Pomelo

Servings: 1 | Prep Time: 10 Minutes

Both of these are nutrient powerhouses. Pomelos contain 600% of your daily requirement of vitamin C, high in fiber, and helps with circulation. Beets, help with digestion, detox the liver and kidneys, and are high in iron.

Ingredients:

1 medium sized beet

2 large pomelo

Directions:

1. Cut up the beet. Peel and segment the pomelos.
2. Juice them in your Omega juicer.

Nutritional Info: Calories: 245 | Sodium: 58 mg | Dietary Fiber: 8.8 g | Total Fat: 0.8 g | Total Carbs: 61.1 g | Protein: 5.4 g.

Blood Orange Chili

Servings: 1 | Prep Time: 12 Minutes

Chilies contain a very powerful anti-inflammatory called capsaicin. Blood oranges contain a phytonutrient called anthocyanins that fights inflammation. Be careful because this is spicy.

Ingredients:

6 blood oranges

2 serrano chili

Agave nectar (optional)

Directions:

1. Peel the oranges. Slice the chilies in half and remove the seeds.

2. Gradually press the ingredients in your Omega juicer.

3. Add agave to sweeten if desired.

Nutritional Info: Calories: 519 | Sodium: 0 mg | Dietary Fiber: 26.6 g | Total Fat: 1.3 g | Total Carbs: 129.8 g | Protein: 10.4 g.

Blueberry Green Juice

Servings: 1 | Prep Time: 5 Minutes

Blueberries are packed with antioxidants that help your overall health. They also contain anti-inflammatory compounds. Spinach is high in vitamin K which boosts memory.

Ingredients:

2 cups fresh blueberries

2 cups fresh spinach leaves

2 fuji apples

Directions:

1. Cut up the apples and remove the seeds. Slice the spinach for about half an inch.

2. Feed the Omega chute alternately with fruits and greens.

Nutritional Info: Calories: 369 | Sodium: 53 mg | Dietary Fiber: 17.1 g | Total Fat: 1.9 g | Total Carbs: 94.5 g | Protein: 4.9 g.

Dill-ightful Glow

Servings: 1 | Prep Time: 7 Minutes

The carrots are packed with antioxidant rich vitamins A&C. The lemon is alkalizing and will help balance your pH. Dill is mineral rich, and its essential oil helps to inhibit bacterial growth.

Ingredients:

1 apple

1 lemon

4 carrots

1 head celery

1 bunch dill

Directions:

1. Cut up the apple and remove the seeds. Peel the lemon. Slice the carrots, celery, and dill.

2. Juice the ingredients in your Omega juicer. Press the dill in between fruits.

Nutritional Info: Calories: 537 | Sodium: 450 mg | Dietary Fiber: 297 g | Total Fat: 6.1 g | Total Carbs: 126.3 g | Protein: 28.7 g.

Full Spectrum Juice

Servings: 2 | Prep Time: 7 Minutes

Broccoli contains a ton of vitamins, minerals, antioxidants, and phytonutrients. It helps with inflammation, cancer prevention, detoxification, and heart health. Ginger has anti-inflammatory, anti-microbial, and antibacterial compounds. Cucumbers are hydrating, and will help remove toxins, and help the cells function better. Lemons are high in vitamin C and are alkalizing.

Ingredients:

1 bell pepper

1 head/stem broccoli

1 lemon

1 cucumber

1 knob ginger

1 tablespoon apple cider vinegar

Directions:

1. Slice the bell pepper, cucumber, and ginger. Peel the lemons and slice into small wedges. Cut up the broccoli.

2. Start to juice the hard produce (broccoli), then lemon, ginger, cucumber, and bell pepper.

3. Add the ACV in your juice for more health benefits.

*Nutritional Info: Calories: 206 | Sodium: 37 mg |
Dietary Fiber: 10.1 g | Total Fat: 2.5 g |
Total Carbs: 44.7 g | Protein: 7.5 g.*

Green Lemonade

Servings: 1-2 | Prep Time: 10 Minutes

Kale is packed with so many vitamins it might as well be a multivitamin in itself. It contains lots of antioxidants too. Lemons are high in vitamin C and alkalizing. Cucumbers are hydrating, and will help you get rid of toxins.

Ingredients:

2 small green apples

1 lemon

1/2 cucumber

6 stalks celery

6 large pieces of kale

1-inch piece of ginger

Directions:

1. Slice up the apple, core it, and remove the seeds. Peel the lemon. Slice the cucumber, celery, ginger and kale.

1. Juice the kale in between other ingredients.

Nutritional Info: Calories: 119 | Sodium: 49 mg | Dietary Fiber: 6.1 g | Total Fat: 0.7 g | Total Carbs: 30.3 g | Protein: 2.1 g.

Hawaiian Morning

Servings: 2 | Prep Time: 10 Minutes

The coconut water provides your body with electrolytes. Think of it as a healthy version of a sports drink. Mango contain anti-inflammatory compounds, and improve the skin. Peaches contain zinc which helps boost the immune system.

Ingredients:

1 cup peaches

1 cup mango

1 fresh orange

1/2 cup coconut water

1 teaspoon agave nectar

Directions:

1.   Slice the peaches and remove the pit. Peel the mango, and cut it into slices. Peel the orange.

2.   Feed the first 3 ingredients in your Omega juicer.

3.   Mix the juice with the coconut water, and agave.

Nutritional Info: Calories: 172 | Sodium: 5 mg | Dietary Fiber: 5.8 g | Total Fat: 7.1 g | Total Carbs: 28.1 g | Protein: 2.4 g.

Pineapple Mango

Servings: 1 | Prep Time: 10 Minutes

Pineapples are high in vitamin C which is good for both skin and the immune system. The bromelain in pineapples is good for digestion. The antioxidants in mangos help prevent cancer. Mangos also aid in digestion, improve eye health and skin. Limes are alkalizing, and contain vitamin C.

Ingredients:

1 firm mango

2 cups pineapple

2 large juicy limes

Directions:

1. Peel, pit, and slice the mango. Chop up the pineapple. Peel the limes.

2. In any order, juice the produce using your Omega juicer.

Nutritional Info: Calories: 274 | Sodium: 9 mg | Dietary Fiber: 10.1 g | Total Fat: 0.9 g | Total Carbs: 74.4 g | Protein: 3.2 g.

Rhubarb carrot

Servings: 1 | Prep Time: 10 Minutes

Rhubarb is packed with tons of nutrients that aid in weight loss, helps with bones, helps prevent Alzheimer's disease, prevents cancer, and stimulates red blood cell production. Rhubarb is very tart so the carrots help sweeten the juice.

Ingredients:

8 large fresh carrots

1 cup rhubarb

1 large fresh mint sprig

1 fresh lemon

Directions:

1. Chop up the rhubarb making sure to discard the stems. Peel the lemon. Slice the carrots, mint, and lemon, about half an inch.

2. Juice in your Omega juicer by pressing the ingredients in the chute. Remember to run the greens in between hard produce.

Nutritional Info: Calories: 283 | Sodium: 406 mg | Dietary Fiber: 18.7 g | Total Fat: 0.5 g | Total Carbs: 68.5 g | Protein: 6.8 g.

Strawberry Cantaloupe

Servings: 1 | Prep Time: 10 Minutes

Cantaloupe as a broad spectrum of vitamins, and antioxidants. Many of the nutrients reside in the rind so don't be shy about using it. Cantaloupe also has anti-inflammatory properties. Strawberries contain anti-inflammatory compounds, and helps reduce plaque on teeth.

Ingredients:

1/4 cantaloupe

4 large strawberries

Directions:

1.   Remove the stems from the strawberries. Slice up the cantaloupe, keeping the rind on.

2.   Feed the Omega juicer with your ingredients.

3.   Chill or put ice cubes to make it more refreshing.

Nutritional Info: Calories: 27 | Sodium: 6 mg | Dietary Fiber: 1.3 g | Total Fat: 0.2 g | Total Carbs: 6.5 g | Protein: 0.6 g.

Sweet Apple and Celery Juice

Servings: 1 | Prep Time: 5 minutes

This juice is jammed packed with good tasting foods that are good for you. This recipe is an anti-inflammatory, antifungal and antioxidant miracle in a glass. The superfoods in this mixture helps to remove toxins from the body while delivering major nutritional value. You will feel great and look great!

Ingredients:

2 sweet apples

3 stalks celery

1 large bunch dandelion greens

2 leaves kale

1-inch ginger (optional)

Directions:

1. Alternately juice the ingredients with fruits and greens. This is to get the optimum juice of greens.

2. Use food pusher to press them through the juicer on high-speed.

3. Drink immediately for highest nutritional value. Store in an airtight container in the refrigerator and drink within three days.

Nutritional Info: Calories: 357 | Sodium: 308 mg |
Dietary Fiber: 21.7 g | Total Fat: 3.1 g |
Total Carbs: 84.3 g | Protein: 10.9 g.

Tomato Juice

Servings: 30 | Prep Time: 30 Minutes

Tomatoes are packed with vitamins, minerals, and the antioxidant lycopene. Tomatoes can improve colon health, digestive problems, lower cholesterol, amongst other things. Lycopene has been shown to lower the risk of various types of cancer.

Ingredients:

1 bushel tomatoes (half Roma and half regular)

Directions:

1. Core the tomatoes
2. Juice the tomatoes on your Omega juicer.

Nutritional Info: Calories: 144 | Sodium: 39 mg | Dietary Fiber: 9.6 g | Total Fat: 1.6 g | Total Carbs: 31.2 g | Protein: 7.0 g.

Watermelon Tomato

Servings: 1 | Prep Time: 7 Minutes

Watermelon is filled with a variety of vitamins and minerals to help your overall health. It is also very hydrating. Tomatoes are high in vitamin C which is good for your immune system, and skin. This is a great summer refresher.

Ingredients:

1/2 small watermelon

2 medium tomatoes

Directions:

1. Cut up the watermelon and remove the seeds. Cut up the tomatoes.

2. In your Omega juicer, feed the chute with the watermelon and tomatoes.

Nutritional Info: Calories: 195 | Sodium: 19 mg | Dietary Fiber: 4.9 g | Total Fat: 1.1 g | Total Carbs: 47.1 g | Protein: 5.1 g.

19

Weight Loss

Bye-Bye Belly

Servings: 1 | Prep Time: 3 minutes

This juice will help you reach your weight loss goals. It gives you the feeling of satisfaction and keeps hunger at bay. As an added benefit is that it naturally speeds up the metabolism. It removes toxins from the body, cleanses the blood and the liver. This juice is very rich in vitamins and nutrients.

Ingredients:

1 cup kale

1 beet

3 carrots

1 apple

Directions:

1. Place kale in through the chute. Use the food pusher to press it into the Omega.

2. Add the beet, carrots and apple to the food chute and juice.

3. Note: if the earthy flavors of the kale and beet is too strong for your taste, you may substitute spinach and 1 cup of dark berries of your choice.

Nutritional Info: Calories: 247 | Sodium: 234 mg | Dietary Fiber: 11.9 g | Total Fat: 0.5 g | Total Carbs: 60.1 g | Protein: 5.7 g.

Kale and Carrot Cocktail

Servings: 2 | Prep Time: 2 minutes

This is energy in a glass! Kale is full of iron, minerals and nutrients. The carrots, grapes, and apple add fiber and crisp sweetness. This combination is a powerful overall health juice. These nutrients are used to fight cancer, enhance eye health and to remove toxins and inflammation of the intestines to prevent many illnesses before they are introduced to the body.

Ingredients:

1 bunch of kale

6 carrots

2 cups red grapes

1 red apple

Directions:

1. Juice the kale, followed by the red grapes on your Omega juicer.

2. Then, process the carrots and apple.

3. This juice can be consumed immediately, or you can allow it to chill in the refrigerator for one hour, then stir and enjoy.

Nutritional Info: Calories: 254 | Sodium: 190 mg | Dietary Fiber: 9.7 g | Total Fat: 0.5 g | Total Carbs: 61.2 g | Protein: 6.6 g.

Metabolism Boost Juice

Servings: 1 | Prep Time: 5 minutes

This light and refreshing juice will boost your metabolic rate while detoxing your system. This super-hydrating recipe has the added bonus of anti-inflammatory properties. You will feel energetic and ready to take on your day after this drink!

Ingredients:

1 cucumber

1 stalk of celery

1-inch of ginger

1-inch turmeric

1/2 lemon

1 cup coconut water

Directions:

1. Pour the coconut water into the juice jug before juicing.
2. Juice all the ingredients in your Omega juicer.

Nutritional Info: Calories: 375 | Sodium: 40 mg | Dietary Fiber: 11.5 g | Total Fat: 28.0 g | Total Carbs: 33.1 g | Protein: 6.0 g.

Papaya Cucumber Juice

Servings: 1 | Prep Time: 6 minutes

Papaya has long been considered the healing fruit. It is full of antioxidants and is great for intestinal and cardiovascular healing. Papaya is combined with hydrating cucumber and crisp apple for a unique and savory blend. This drink is flavored with all natural honey, fresh mint, and cinnamon. This vitamin-rich and mineral-packed juice can also be added to your cleansing regimen.

Ingredients:

1 green (unripen) papaya

1 green apple

1 cucumber

1 cup mint

1 teaspoon raw honey

1 teaspoon ground cinnamon

Directions:

1. Peel the green (unripen) papaya, cut in half and remove the seeds. Place the papaya and the cucumber into the chute together, directly followed by the green apple. Juice the mint in between.

2. Use the food pusher to press them into the Omega Juicer.

3. Add the raw honey and ground cinnamon to the juice jug after juice is prepared.

4. Stir and serve. This juice can be stored in an airtight container and kept refrigerated for 12 hours. Stir juice before serving each time.

Nutritional Info: Calories: 342 | Sodium: 62 mg |
Dietary Fiber: 18.8 g | Total Fat: 2.2 g |
Total Carbs: 85.4 g | Protein: 7.1 g.

20

Energy

Bootroot Zinger

Servings: 1 | Prep Time: 5 Minutes

Beetroots give your body slow releasing energy that will last a long time. Ginger gives a nice burst of energy, and contains anti-inflammatory compounds.

Ingredients:

2 apples

1 large beet

1-inch piece ginger

Directions:

1.   Slice the apples, core them, and remove the seeds. Cut up the beet and slice ginger.

2.   Feed all the ingredients in your Omega chute until all become dried pulp.

Nutritional Info: Calories: 238 | Sodium: 59 mg | Dietary Fiber: 10.9 g | Total Fat: 1.1 g | Total Carbs: 60.8 g | Protein: 2.6 g.

Energy Juice

Servings: 1 | Prep Time: 7 Minutes

Oranges provide long lasting energy with help from its pectin. Lemons help oxygenate the cells which also provides energy.

Ingredients:

1 orange

4 carrots

1/2 lemon

1/4-inch fresh ginger root

2-3 mint leaves

Directions:

1. Peel and slice the ingredients for about half an inch to fit into the chute.

2. Using your Omega juicer, place the produce in the chute and start to juice.

Nutritional Info: Calories: 216 | Sodium: 172 mg | Dietary Fiber: 12.2 g | Total Fat: 0.7 g | Total Carbs: 52.6 g | Protein: 4.7 g.

High Energy Juice

Servings: 2 | Prep Time: 10 Minutes

Beetroots give your body slow releasing energy that helps increase stamina. Celery and cucumbers are both hydrating which will also boost energy. Apples beneficial fiber and vitamin profile also provide a jolt of energy.

Ingredients:

1 beet

6 celery stalks

1 green apple

1/2 cucumber

Directions:

1. Chop up the beet. Slice the apple, remove the core and seeds. Wash the beet thoroughly, peel and slice into quarter.

2. Juice slowly on your Omega juicer.

Nutritional Info: Calories: 89 | Sodium: 82 mg |
Dietary Fiber: 4.4 g | Total Fat: 0.4 g |
Total Carbs: 21.8 g | Protein: 1.9 g.

Heart Health

Servings: 1 | Prep Time: 10 Minutes

Apples contain antioxidants and phytonutrients that reduce the risk of heart disease. Pears are a great source of fiber which can help lower cholesterol. Carrots are high in vitamin C, which lowers your risk of coronary heart disease.

Ingredients:

4-5 large carrots

1 medium apple

1 pear

1/4-inch fresh ginger

Directions:

1. Slice, core, and remove the seeds from the apple and pear. Slice carrots and ginger.

2. Juice all ingredients on your Omega juicer.

Nutritional Info: Calories: 327 | Sodium: 252 mg | Dietary Fiber: 17.7 g | Total Fat: 0.6 g | Total Carbs: 82.7 g | Protein: 4.1 g.

Orange Coconut

Servings: 1 | Prep Time: 10 Minutes

Coconut water has been shown to lower blood pressure, cholesterol, and triglyceride levels. Coconut water has also been shown to aid in recovery after a heart attack. Oranges are high in vitamin C, which lowers your risk of coronary heart disease.

Ingredients:

1 large young coconut

2 oranges

Directions:

1. Peel and segment the oranges. Cut open the coconut and pour the clear liquid into a glass. Discard any debris in the liquid.

2. Juice the oranges.

3. Pour the coconut water into the same glass as the orange juice, and mix.

Nutritional Info: Calories: 456 | Sodium: 16 mg | Dietary Fiber: 16.0 g | Total Fat: 27.2 g | Total Carbs: 55.4 g | Protein: 6.2 g.

Super Energy

Servings: 1-2 | Prep Time: 12 Minutes

This juice is great way to start your day. It's an alternative to coffee. The secret is the sweet potato which contains complex carbs that will give you energy throughout the day.

Ingredients:

1 sweet potato

1 yellow squash

3 large carrots

1 large apple

Directions:

1. Slice the apple, core it, and remove the seeds. Cut up the yellow squash and sweet potato. Slice the carrots.

2. Slowly feed the Omega chute starting with the potato and finishing with the apple.

Nutritional Info: Calories: 169 | Sodium: 106 mg | Dietary Fiber: 8.3 g | Total Fat: 0.5 g | Total Carbs: 41.1 g | Protein: 3.5 g.

The Energizer

Servings: 4 | Prep Time: 10 Minutes

Coconut water contains electrolytes that provide your body with energy. Apples contain pectin which gives you sustained energy.

Ingredients:

2 pints pineapple

2 pints watermelon

2 quarts coconut water

1 bunch spinach

1-2 cups blueberries

2 green apples

Directions:

1. Slice the apples, core them, and remove the seeds. Slice all other ingredients, about half an inch, except for blueberries.

2. Use your Omega juicer to juice all the ingredients listed. Juice the spinach in between fruits.

3. Mix the juice with the coconut water.

Nutritional Info: Calories: 802 | Sodium: 104 mg | Dietary Fiber: 23.1 g | Total Fat: 54.6 g | Total Carbs: 83.6 g | Protein: 10.4 g.

The Revitalizer

Servings: 2 | Prep Time: 10 Minutes

Kale has a wide variety of vitamins and minerals that fuel the body with energy. Cucumbers provide hydration for the cells and increase energy.

Ingredients:

2 large tomatoes

1 large cucumber

2 apples

2 branches of kale

Directions:

1. Cut up the tomatoes. Slice the apples, core them, and remove the seeds. Slice cucumber and kale for about half an inch.

2. Place the ingredients in your Omega juicer one at a time. Use the food pusher to press the ingredients through the juicer.

Nutritional Info: Calories: 164 | Sodium: 26 mg | Dietary Fiber: 7.8 g | Total Fat: 0.9 g | Total Carbs: 40.6 g | Protein: 3.9 g.

21

For Kids

Kid's Veggie Juice

Servings: 1 | Prep Time: 10 Minutes

This juice is a great way to get your kids to eat their vegetables without them knowing it. Beets have a wide spectrum of vitamins, minerals, and phytonutrients. Spinach is packed with calcium and iron. The pineapple and apple give this a sweet taste kids love, while providing vitamin C, and healthy pectin.

Ingredients:

1 small beetroot

2 apples

1/4 small pineapple

1 stick of celery

1 small handful of spinach

1-inch slice of cucumber

Directions:

1. Cut up the pineapple and beet. Slice the apples, core them, and remove the seeds. Slice the spinach, cucumber, and celery.

2. Alternately place the ingredients into Omega juicer.

Nutritional Info: Calories: 106 | Sodium: 73 mg | Dietary Fiber: 5.5 g | Total Fat: 0.6 g | Total Carbs: 25.7 g | Protein: 3.2 g.

Orange Cleanser Juice

Servings: 1 | Prep Time: 3 minutes

This juice is so delicious; your kids will not know it is good for them. Sweet carrots, celery, oranges, and a little ginger make a healthy, kid-pleasing drink. Loaded with fiber, vitamin C and magnesium; Orange Cleanser Juice is great for the skin, helps fight off colds and aids in digestion and keeps eyes healthy.

Ingredients:

2 oranges

2 carrots

2 stalks of celery

1-inch ginger

Directions:

1. Peel the oranges and place into the food chute of your Omega Juicer. Follow the next three ingredients.

2. Use the food pusher to press the fruit into the juicer.

3. Put the remaining foods into the food chute and repeat the process, with the juicer settings adjusted to high-speed. Pour and serve.

Nutritional Info: Calories: 247 | Sodium: 113 mg | Dietary Fiber: 13.1 g | Total Fat: 0.8 g | Total Carbs: 60.1 g | Protein: 5.2 g.

Tomato Carrot

Servings: 3 | Prep Time: 10 Minutes

This is a deliciously sweet juice that kids will love. It's packed with vitamins A & C, as well as tons of antioxidants. It also contains lutein and lycopene which are good for eye health. Lutein helps with exercise related asthma as well.

Ingredients:

6 medium carrots

2 tomatoes

2 oranges

1 grapefruit

Directions:

1.   Peel the grapefruit, and oranges. Cut up the tomatoes. Slice the carrots.

2.   Slowly feed the ingredients into the Omega chute.

Nutritional Info: Calories: 136 | Sodium: 88 mg | Dietary Fiber: 7.4 g | Total Fat: 0.3 g | Total Carbs: 33.1 g | Protein: 3.1 g.

22

For Athletes

Athlete's Super Fuel

Servings: 3-4 | Prep Time: 10 Minutes

Drink this before or after a workout. The watermelon is hydrating and will help replace the water lost after a workout. The manganese found in pineapple regulates blood sugar, and fights free radicals.

Ingredients:

1/2 watermelon

1 lemon

5 oranges

1 can pineapple concentrate, frozen

Directions:

1. Thaw the pineapple. Peel the lemon, and oranges. Cut up the watermelon into cubes.

2. Juice the ingredients in your Omega juicer.

3. Mix the juice with the concentrate.

Nutritional Info: Calories: 149 | Sodium: 2 mg |
Dietary Fiber: 7.6 g | Total Fat: 0.5 g |
Total Carbs: 38.5 g | Protein: 3.1 g.

Joggers Paradise

Servings: 1 | Prep Time: 10 Minutes

This is great to drink while you're on a run. It contains natural sugar that will give you quick energy. The complex carbs in the yams will give you long term energy and stamina. The vitamin C and vitamin A from the fruit will fight free radicals and help with recovery.

Ingredients:

3 oranges

2 hard pears

1 small yam

Directions:

1. Peel the pears, Core them, and remove the seeds. Peel the oranges and yam; slice them for about quarter of an inch.

2. Juice the produce in your Omega juicer.

Nutritional Info: Calories: 580 | Sodium: 10 mg | Dietary Fiber: 28.9 g | Total Fat: 1.4 g | Total Carbs: 142.2 g | Protein: 7.7 g.

23

Brain

The Brain Stimulator

Servings: 1 | Prep Time: 10 Minutes

The flavonoids in oranges and grapefruit improve brain functions such as memory. The carotenoids in sweet potatoes help support cognitive function.

Ingredients:

1 orange

1 hard pear

1 sweet potato

1 grapefruit

1 apple

Directions:

1.   Peel the oranges and sweet potatoes (slice into cubes). Slice, core, and remove the seeds from the apples and pears. Peel grapefruit.

2.   Fill the Omega chute with the ingredients listed. Press the chute using the food pusher to get more juice.

Nutritional Info: Calories: 406 | Sodium: 44 mg |
Dietary Fiber: 18.4 g | Total Fat: 1.1 g |
Total Carbs: 101.9 g | Protein: 5.8 g.

Cognitive Power Up

Servings: 1 | Prep Time: 7 minutes

Beets are a natural vasodilator that help improve blood flow to the brain. The carotenoids in sweet potatoes help support cognitive function, and the complex carbs give you sustained energy. Luteolin in carrots has been shown to reduce age-related memory issues, and brain inflammation.

Ingredients:

1 beetroot

1 sweet potato

3 medium carrots

Directions:

1. Chop up the beetroot. Slice the sweet potato into small cubes or strips.

2. Juice all ingredients on your Omega juicer.

Nutritional Info: Calories: 222 | Sodium: 244 mg | Dietary Fiber: 10.3 g | Total Fat: 0.4 g | Total Carbs: 51.6 g | Protein: 5.5 g.

24

Mood

Destress Juice

Servings: 1 | Prep Time: 12 Minutes

The vitamin C in the lemon helps reduce the stress hormone cortisol. The B vitamins in spinach help with stress management, anxiety, and depression. The phosphorus, and iron in apples helps to fight against the oxidizing effects of stress.

Ingredients:

1/2 honeydew melon

100 g baby Spinach

2 (410g) apples

1/2 lemon

Directions:

1. Cut up the honeydew. Slice the apples, core them, and remove the seeds. Peel the lemon and slice. De-stem the spinach.

2. Juice the produce using the Omega juicer. Run the spinach in between fruits.

Nutritional Info: Calories: 430 | Sodium: 173 mg | Dietary Fiber: 17.2 g | Total Fat: 1.9 g | Total Carbs: 109.8 g | Protein: 7.0 g.

Mood Booster

Beets are great mood boosters with magnesium that calms nerves, and tryptophan that enhances and stabilizes mood. Blueberries contain anthocyanin which has been shown to boost people's mood.

Ingredients:

3 ribs celery

1/2 small beet

1 cup blueberries

Directions:

1. Cut up the beet.
2. Juice the blueberries first, then the other hard ingredients.

Nutritional Info: Calories: 107 | Sodium: 48 mg | Dietary Fiber: 4.7 g | Total Fat: 0.6 g | Total Carbs: 26.3 g | Protein: 2.0 g.

Tropical Citrus Delight

Servings: 1 | Prep Time: 15 Minutes

This refreshing juice can help with anxiety and stress. The vitamin C in oranges lowers the stress hormone cortisol. Peaches contain a natural sedative to help keep you calm.

Ingredients:

1 medium coconut

2 large oranges

2 medium peaches

Directions:

1. Remove the meat from the coconut and discard the rest. Peel the oranges. Slice up the peaches and remove the pit.

2. Feed the Omega chute with the ingredients listed.

Nutritional Info: Calories: 165 | Sodium: 79 mg | Dietary Fiber: 47.5 g | Total Fat: 133.5 g | Total Carbs: 122.3 g | Protein: 18.7 g.

25

Hormones

Carrot Pineapple Turmeric Spritzer

Servings: 1 | Prep Time: 7 Minutes

This is great for women during the worst parts of their cycle. The bromelain in pineapple is a great anti-inflammatory and helps with cramps. The manganese in pineapples helps with irritability, mood swings, and headaches. Turmeric contains anti-inflammatory, anti-depressant, and pain killing properties. Carrots help the body remove the excess estrogen that happens during this part of the cycles.

Ingredients:

1/4 of a large pineapple, making sure to include all or part of the core

2-3 large carrots

1/8 – 1/4 teaspoon turmeric powder

Sparkling mineral water

Directions:

1. Cut up the pineapple and include the core. Slice the carrots.

2. Slowly feed the Omega chute with pineapple and carrots.

3. Mix in the turmeric, and top off with sparkling water.

Nutritional Info: Calories: 110 | Sodium: 149 mg | Dietary Fiber: 6.0 g | Total Fat: 0.1 g | Total Carbs: 26.9 g | Protein: 2.0 g.

Next Steps...

DID YOU ENJOY THE BOOK?

IF SO, THEN LET ME KNOW BY LEAVING A REVIEW ON AMAZON! Reviews are the lifeblood of independent authors. I would appreciate even a few words and rating if that's all you have time for. Here's the link:

http://www.healthyhappyfoodie.org/s2-freebooks

IF YOU DID NOT LIKE THIS BOOK, THEN PLEASE TELL ME! Email me at feedback@HHFpress.com and let me know what you didn't like! Perhaps I can change it. In today's world a book doesn't have to be stagnant, it can improve with time and feedback from readers like you. You can impact this book, and I welcome your feedback. Help make this book better for everyone!

DO YOU LIKE FREE BOOKS?

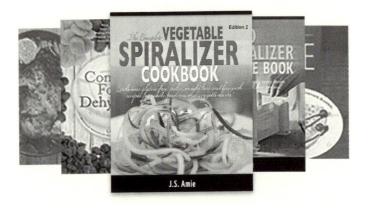

Every month we release a new book, and we offer it to our current readers first...absolutely free! This helps us get early feedback before launching a book, and lets you stock your shelf full of interesting and valuable books for free!

Some recent titles include:

- The Complete Vegetable Spiralizer Cookbook
- My Lodge Cast Iron Skillet Cookbook
- 101 The New Crepes Cookbook

To receive this month's free book, just go to

http://www.healthyhappyfoodie.org/s2-freebooks

.

Made in the USA
Columbia, SC
20 January 2018